Mediterranean Diet Cookbook for Beginners

The Ultimate Beginner's Mediterranean Diet Kickstart Guide. Easy Meal Plan & Proven Heart Healthy Recipes. Everything You Need to Know to Get Started Today!

By*Abigail Murphy*

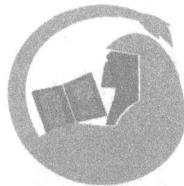

EFFINGO
Publishing

I0135295

For more great books, visit:

EffingoPublishing.com

Download another book for Free

We want to thank you for purchasing this book and offer you another book (just as long and valuable as this book), "Health & Fitness Mistakes You Don't Know You're Making," completely free.

Visit the link below to signup and receive it:

www.effingopublishing.com/gift

In this book, we will break down the most common health & fitness mistakes, you are probably committing right now, and will reveal how you can quickly get in the best shape of your life!

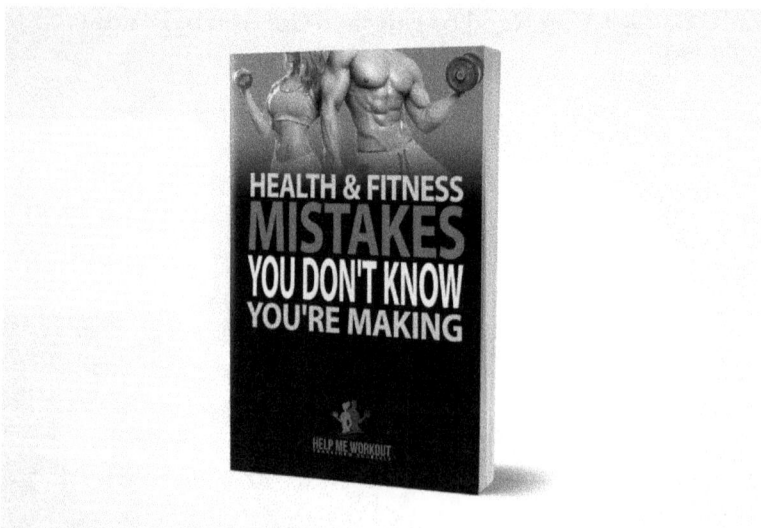

In addition to this valuable gift, you will also have an opportunity to get our new books for free, enter giveaways, and receive other useful emails from us. Again, visit the link to sign up:

www.effingopublishing.com/gift

TABLE OF CONTENTS

INTRODUCTION

You are what you eat. The choices you make concerning what you put on your plate ultimately defines the kind of life you enjoy. So how about making a switch to Mediterranean?

The Mediterranean Lifestyle is more than just the food; it is a way of life. This Mediterranean Diet Cookbook for Beginners will equip you with strategies that will make your journey and transition, smooth and relatively easy. More than a cookbook, this will be your ultimate guide and partner towards victory. It will include over fifty (50) recipes that are easy-to-follow and a 2-week meal plan to get you started on the right path.

"A healthy diet is a solution to
many of our health-care
problems. It's the most
important solution."

John Mackey

They always say you are what you eat. Your choices on the plate, ultimately, define the kind of life you enjoy. So what's on your plate? Are you eating healthily enough? Whether you're willing to make amends because you want to lose weight or you wish to be healthier, you have made the right decision to pick up this book.

This Mediterranean Diet Cookbook for Beginners is a perfect guide for anyone starting. It will contain everything you need to get started, including recipes for you to try, and a two-week meal plan to direct your path accordingly. This book is also equipped with easy-to-follow tips and strategies to make your journey more worthwhile.

Starting a new diet can be quite daunting. Breaking through your routine is not going to be simple, but it is not impossible. The Mediterranean Diet Cookbook for Beginners aims to make the journey more promising, by equipping you with strategies that will guarantee ease of execution and overall success. More than a cookbook, this will be your ultimate guide and partner towards victory.

Also, before you get started, I recommend you **joining our email newsletter** to receive updates on any upcoming new book releases or promotions. You can sign-up for free, and as a bonus, you will receive a gift. Our *"Health & Fitness Mistakes You Don't Know You're Making"* book! This book has been written to demystify, expose the top do's and don'ts and to finally equip you with the information you need to get in the best shape of your life. Due to the overwhelming amount of misinformation and lies told by magazines and self-proclaimed "gurus," it's becoming harder and harder to get reliable information to get in shape. You don't have to go through dozens of biased, unreliable, and untrustworthy sources to get your health & fitness information. Everything you need to help you has been broken down in this book for you to easily follow and to immediately get results to achieve your desired fitness goals in the shortest amount of time.

Once again, to join our free email newsletter and to receive a free copy of this valuable book, please visit the link and signup now: **www.effingopublishing.com/gift**

CHAPTER 1: WHAT IS MEDITERRANEAN DIET?

The roots of Mediterranean Cuisine cannot be credited to a single country or culture. But the world's earliest civilizations that surrounded the Mediterranean Sea. Through the trades that happened, this diet proves to be a massive collaboration between Europe, Asia, and Africa.

The climate around these areas contributes to the cuisine's characteristic warmth and sunny feel. It involves the use of a lot of fruits, vegetables, whole grains, nuts, beans, and seeds. Olive oil is the most prominent ingredient since olive trees are abundant in the area. Apart from its health benefits, it gives the dishes a unique punchy, fermented, and acidic taste.

The worldwide interest in Mediterranean Diet did not come until the 1960s. During that time, there was a noted rise in deaths related to heart disease, but levels were considerably lower in the Mediterranean countries. Since then, this diet has been recommended for dietary guidelines to patients suffering from heart disease; and it is highly recognized by the World Health Organization (WHO) because of its sustainability.

Benefits of the Mediterranean Diet

There is a myriad of diet options available for everyone. These choices can be quite overwhelming, so it is common for people to plunge into diet fads that only seem promising on the surface, but does not offer considerable value.

A beginner Mediterranean diet is more than a weight loss program. When appropriately implemented, it is a transformative lifestyle that can improve and enhance your existence.

To better understand it, here is a detailed discussion on the benefits of adopting a Mediterranean lifestyle:

1. **It keeps the muscles strong and agile.** It is natural for the body to deteriorate with age slowly. With the prolonged observance of the Mediterranean Diet, you will see a significant decrease in muscle weakness and frailty so that you will remain active and agile even with age.

2. **It prevents the onset of heart disease and stroke.** The heart-healthy benefits of the Mediterranean Diet are due to the exclusion of processed food, red meat, refined bread, and hard liquor from the diet. The lifestyle takes better consideration of what you eat, so your heart is protected from harm. Studies show that patients who switched to a Mediterranean Diet rich in nuts and extra virgin olive oil saw a 30% decrease in heart attack episodes and a 20% decrease in stroke incidents.

3. **It helps control the progression and development of Type 2 Diabetes.** Mediterranean Diet is fiber-rich, and so it aids in digestion and metabolism. With proper implementation, a patient can effectively control spikes in his blood sugar levels, allowing healthy control over Diabetes. More importantly, it helps in weight loss.

4. **It lowers the risk of developing Alzheimer's Disease.** Alzheimer's Disease is a degenerative disease that involves brain cells. It is progressive, and when a person has Alzheimer's Disease, one's mental, social, and behavioral skills are affected. The risk of Alzheimer's Disease and Dementia is reduced with improved cholesterol, circulation, and blood sugar levels

5. It also lowers the risk of developing Parkinson's Disease. Mediterranean Diet is rich in antioxidants from fruits, vegetables, and healthy fats. Maintenance of this kind of diet prevents oxidative stress that will bring damage, and so cause degeneration related to Parkinson's Disease.

6. It helps reduce inflammation. Studies show that a prolonged observance of the Mediterranean Diet can significantly reduce the rate of inflammation bio-markers that bring about chronic suffering. Oxidative stress is the root cause of inflammation, but the high levels of antioxidants in the Mediterranean Diet will help control the onset of inflammation. Foods rich in betaine (spinach, beets) and choline (soybeans, egg yolks) have increased anti-inflammatory properties.

7. **It helps combat cancer.** Research has shown that adherence to a Mediterranean Lifestyle helps in reducing the risk of cancer development, as well as cancer-related mortality.

8. **It improves skin condition.** Olive oil is rich in Vitamin E and antioxidants, and red wine is rich in resveratrol that inhibits the growth bacteria. Prolonged intake of the Mediterranean Diet will cause your skin to appear more radiant and glowing.

9. **It prolongs life.** With the continued implementation of the Mediterranean Diet, you protect your heart from heart disease, cancer, and all kinds of illnesses. This kind of protection prolongs life by significantly reducing the risk of death by 20%.

10. **It aids in weight loss.** The Mediterranean Diet is low in calories, and this helps in weight loss. To lose weight, people struggle with calorie-counting, as a means to control their food intake. The basic ingredients of the Mediterranean Diet are low in calories, so you don't have to bother counting. They are also fiber-rich, so this diet helps improve digestion.

11. Contrary to what many people think, weight loss is not about starving yourself. It is about eating right and choosing the right ingredients. By observing this diet, you can start celebrating impressive weight loss gains.

CHAPTER 2: GETTING STARTED ON YOUR DIET

The misconception about the Mediterranean Diet is that it is about eating fresh and raw food. Knowledge of the Mediterranean Diet Pyramid will teach you that the dinner table is not limit to fruits and vegetables. Although they make up the most significant component of this diet, there is so much more to Mediterranean meals than just fruits and vegetables.

Your Mediterranean Diet Shopping List: Your Way Around the Mediterranean Kitchen

What makes up the Mediterranean Diet Pyramid? To better appreciate this diet and what you are going to be dealing with, in the kitchen, here is an overview of your typical Mediterranean shopping list.

Fruits& Vegetables. The bulk of the Mediterranean Diet is all about fruits and vegetables. They are low in calories and are rich in all kinds of vitamins and minerals. Your shopping list should include more of the following:

a. Fruits (apples, apricots, avocado, bananas, berries, cherries, clementines, dates, figs, grapes, melons, oranges, pears, peaches, strawberries, tomatoes)

b. Vegetables (artichokes, arugula, beets, broccoli, Brussel sprouts, cabbage, cauliflower, collard greens, cucumbers, kale, onions, peas, peppers, potatoes, spinach, turnips, yams, zucchini)

Oils. Olive oil is the primary source of healthy fats in Mediterranean meals. It contains monosaturated fat, which lowers cholesterol and the so-called bad fats (LDL). You may use olive oils for cooking, and it may serve as a salad dressing.

Nuts, Seeds, Grains, and Legumes. Nut, like oils, are an excellent source of monosaturated fat. Sources under this category include:

a. Nuts (almonds, cashews, hazelnuts, macadamia nuts, pine nuts, walnuts)

b. Grains (barley, brown rice, bulgur, buckwheat, couscous, farro, wheat berries, whole-grain bread, and wraps)

c. Seeds (sesame, sunflower, pumpkin)

d. Beans and Legumes (chickpeas, fava beans, peanuts, peas, pulses)

Herbs and Spices. Mediterranean dishes are made delicious by a variety of herbs and spices. Among the spices featured are basil, cinnamon, coriander, cilantro, rosemary, mint,oregano, parsley, pepper, sage, tarragon, garlic and so much more. All these spices come with their nutritional benefits.

Fish and Seafood. Fatty fish are rich in omega-3 fatty acids, and they are considered the cornerstone of the Mediterranean Diet. Omega-3 fatty acids are abundant in poly-saturated fat, which has anti-inflammatory properties. Regular intake of Omega-3 fatty acid-rich foods helps to reduce levels of triglycerides and reduce the risk of blood clotting, heart failure, and stroke.Examples of this include the following:

a. Albacore tuna

b. Lake trout

c. Herring

d. Mackerel

e. Salmon

f. Sardines

g. Other seafood (shrimps, shellfish, clams)

Poultry and Eggs. Next to fish, poultry (chicken duck and turkey) would be a good source of healthy protein. Lean meats are consumed in Mediterranean Diets but only in strict moderation.

Meats. Just like fish and poultry, meats are a good source of protein but enjoyed less than poultry. Examples of meats are pork, beef, and lamb.

Cheese and Yogurt. Dairy products allowed in a Mediterranean Diet.

a. Dairy products (unprocessed cheeses such as brie, feta, parmesan, ricotta)

b. Yogurt (plain and Greek yogurt)

Wine. Wine is a prominent feature in Mediterranean cuisine but in strict moderation. This restriction is at about 3-oz for females and 5-oz for males. Wine elevates overall food experience. If the pairing is superb, it can even bring out the flavors of the dish, more effectively.

Preparing for a New Diet: How to Ensure Success

As with every endeavor, it is natural for you to want to claim success over this. Your efforts will be for nothing if you won't be victorious, so you must equip yourself with a plan. To adequately prepare yourself physically, mentally, and socially, the following tips are going to be helpful:

Take it a step-at-a-time. While it would be nice to tackle this in an overnight fashion, it's not going to happen that way. It is going to be hard, and you may stumble a few times before you achieve anything. It's really about applying the right strategy. You can start by having one vegetarian meal per week, and then per day until you can manage a diet that's more Mediterranean.

Cook your food.

The genuine Mediterranean lifestyle involves having a good relationship with the food on your plate. The best way to ensure that is for you to take part in food preparation and cooking. In the kitchen, you will get to know every ingredient and appreciate every detail in the simple dish. This kind of relationship with your food will help you embrace the diet with much ease. Moreover, if you're having fun in the kitchen, then it can be expected that you will have fun while you dine.

1. **Assign healthy substitutes to your usual.** Starting is going to be a challenge, primarily if you're used to all the "bad" food. The following are some appropriate substitutes that you can apply:

Pretzels, chips, crackers and ranch dip →
Carrots, broccoli, and celery with fresh salsa

Stir-fry meat with white rice → Stir-fry vegetables with quinoa

White bread sandwich → Whole wheat tortilla wraps

Ice cream → Non-fat pudding

2. Restructure your kitchen pantry.

Look at your pantry. How is it looking? You have seen the Mediterranean grocery list, so you know what's good and bad for you. Given what you have learned, you should go shopping for brand-new ingredients and get rid of all the food and ingredients that will conflict with the diet you are trying to adopt.

3. Embrace the variety. Mediterranean

Cuisine is not tied to a single country or culture. Its history is vast because it has influences from various countries around the Mediterranean Sea. To properly elevate your dining experience, you have to embrace the variety of dishes that are made available to you. The Mediterranean Diet features dishes with Turkish, Moroccan, Spanish, Italian, Greek, and Middle Eastern roots. Go ahead, expand your palate.

4. Read the label. In the beginning, it may be a

little hard and confusing to shop for ingredients, but

do not be disheartened. You may have been buying food a certain way. After restructuring your pantry, you will be filling it up with new stuff. Reading the labels on the food you buy will help you get to know them more.

5. Enjoy more fish. If you're craving meat, understand that the diet is not exclusively vegetarian. If you are craving for more meaty protein sources, it is safer to choose fish. It is rich in healthy omega-3 fatty acids and is low in calories.

6. Satisfy the holistic Mediterranean Diet Pyramid. Beyond the food, the genuine Mediterranean lifestyle encourages a holistic approach that involves exercise and socialization. It serves as the foundation of the pyramid. Physical activity will enhance the effect of your healthy diet. By engaging in physical activity, you can control your weight loss and metabolism; and with a healthy social life, your Mediterranean lifestyle takes a whole different level. When you have friends and family to support you, the entire journey becomes more fruitful.

Mediterranean Diet FAQs

Before you embark on the actual journey, you may have lingering questions about the diet. Feel free to peruse of this section:

- **Is the Mediterranean Diet going to be expensive to sustain?**

  All diet transitions will cost you some money. You are going to build a new pantry, and you're going to adopt a new lifestyle. In reality, a Mediterranean lifestyle is inexpensive, especially compared to a kitchen pantry that's packed with processed food. The main bulk of the Mediterranean shopping list consists of vegetables, fruits, wheat, and grains.

- **Are pasta and bread good?**

Mediterranean dishes make use of pasta and bread, but servings are limited to a 1 cup or ½ cup (often a side dish). So basically, pasta and bread are good, but you have to define what you enjoy on a plate. To be on the safe side, you should choose products made from whole grains. Stay away from white flour.

- **Is the Mediterranean Diet vegetarian?**

While it appears predominantly vegetarian, it is not. What this diet promotes and teaches is discipline and moderation, so that you can comply with the following components:

a. Daily intake of fruits, vegetables, healthy fats, and grains

b. Weekly consumption of poultry, beans, eggs, poultry, and fish

c. Moderate intake of various dairy products

d. Limited to little or no intake of red meat

- **Is fat forbidden?**

  As already mentioned earlier in the book, olive oil is one of the core ingredients in Mediterranean Cuisine. Its abundance in the Mediterranean Sea has brought about its prominence in the kitchen. Fat is not at all bad, as long as you have the right kind of fat. The fat that's abundant in processed food is extremely unhealthy. These are called trans fats (trans-unsaturated fatty acids), and they are unsaturated. They are found to increase levels of LDL (bad fat) and decrease levels of HDL (good fat) in the body.

- **How many glasses of wine are considered healthy and safe?**

  Always when the subject is alcohol, you have to keep things in moderation. A glass or two of wine per day is safe and healthy, but you have to understand that going over the healthy limit will put your heart in danger.

- **What food or substances should I avoid?**

The Mediterranean Diet is not entirely restrictive. It demands discipline and instills responsibility. However, one should be smart enough to avoid all these unhealthy foods:

a. Processed meats and other processed food (hotdogs, sausages)

b. Refined oils and grains (cottonseed oil, canola oil, soybean oil)

c. Sugar (soda, candy, ice cream)

d. Trans fats (margarine)

- **Is the Mediterranean Diet safe?**

In the rise of several fad diets, it is quite hard to trust that "diets" are meant for long-lasting good. First of all, the Mediterranean Diet is not a fad. It is a lifestyle, and it has been observed by various nations since before it became known between the 1950s and 1960s. This diet is safe because it focusses on the quality of the food and not the quantity. Mediterranean dishes are balanced, so you do not lack anything. More importantly, it improves the general state of your life.

- **Is it okay for me to have coffee?**

Coffee does not go against the restrictions of the diet. The Mediterranean region is obsessed with coffee—especially since it is a potent antioxidant. You have to be more conscious about the coffee you enjoy. Go for brewed coffee or espresso. Enjoy it black and with the least amount of sugar, if possible.

CHAPTER 3: 52 EASY & PROVEN HEART-HEALTHY MEDITERRANEAN DIET RECIPES

Whether you're adopting this new lifestyle for health purposes or you are doing this to lose weight, these Mediterranean Diet Cookbook is going to help you get started. The ingredients and the manner of cooking are characteristic of the Mediterranean Diet. Weight loss is possible because dishes are low in calories, and components are healthy.

In this chapter, you will gain access to simple yet healthy and delicious Mediterranean Diet Recipes. You do not have to be kitchen savvy to tackle them; you have to be willing to make a change in your life. Are you ready?

Breakfasts

The first meal you have in the morning is the most important because it will kickstart your day. You must start things right because it will ultimately determine how the rest of the day will go. You have to place closer attention to whatever you're putting on your plate in the morning because the vitamins and nutrients you have for breakfast will help you function efficiently and effectively throughout the day.

No matter how busy you may be, you have to grab something to eat. Do not skip breakfast because the health ramifications of skipping meals are only going to take a toll on your body and your overall health.

Egg and Quinoa Bowl

Do you know that the combination of nutrient-rich egg yolk and fresh vegetables can increase the absorption of carotenoids in the body? Carotenoids can be your protection against heart disease. So enjoy this tasty bowl, and rest assured that every bite is going to be good for your heart.

Calories	Protein	Carbohydrates	Fat
366	14	33	21

Ingredients:

- ¼ ripe avocado

- 1 egg, brought to room temperature

- ½ tsp garlic, minced

- 1 cup kale, chopped

- 1 ½ tsp olive oil, divided

- ½ cup quinoa, cooked

- 1/3 cup cherry tomatoes, halved

- salt and pepper, to taste

Instructions:

1. In a saucepan boil the egg in about 3 inches water. Do this for just 6 minutes and immediately transfer the egg to ice water and leave it there for 1 minute. Remove the shell and set it aside.

2. In a skillet, sauté garlic. Add kale and stir everything until softened.

3. In a bowl, bring together the sautéed kale, tomatoes, quinoa, and avocado. Drizzle it with ½ tsp olive oil. Season it with salt and pepper to taste.

4. Cut the egg in half, and top everything with the soft-boiled egg.

Mediterranean Scones

What is your ideal morning ritual? Perhaps you want to have a quick sit down with a cuppa. Maybe a tea or a coffee? Now what's perfect with this hot cup is a good scone. This recipe is amazing. It is healthy and delicious.

Calories	Protein	Carbohydrates	Fat
293	8	36	14

Ingredients:

- 1 tbsp baking powder

- 50g butter

- 100g feta cheese, cubed

- 1 egg, beaten

- 350g self-raising flour

- 300ml milk

- 10 black olives, pitted and halved

- 1 tbsp olive oil

- ¼ tsp salt

- 8 sundried tomatoes, chopped

Instructions:

1. Preheat oven to 200°C. Grease a baking sheet.

2. In a bowl, bring together the baking powder, flour, and salt.

3. Add the oil and butter and mix everything until the mixture appears like crumbs.

4. Add the cheese, tomatoes, and olives. Mix everything, then create a well in the center then pour the milk in it. Mix everything, and you should get a sticky dough, but do not overhandle it.

5. Put some flour in your hands and then shape the dough, round. Brush the surface with the egg. Pop the dish into the oven and let it bake until the scones are golden or about 20 minutes.

6. Serve warm with a side of butter.

Bean and Feta Toast

Here's a tasty and fancy baguette recipe with bean and feta cheese. It's not a common combination; the flavors in this recipe makes for a great breakfast experience. Who said your mornings have to be boring? This Mediterranean baguette is fantastic!

Calories	Protein	Carbohydrates	Fat
354	20	28	18

Ingredients:

- 4 slices baguette

- 350g broad bean

- 100g feta cheese, drained

- 1 tsp lemon juice

- 2 tbsp mint leaves, chopped

- 1 tbsp extra virgin olive oil

- 50g mixed salad greens

- 10 cherry tomatoes, halved

Instructions:

1. In a small pan, bring water to boil.

2. Add the beans and let it boil, then drain and run cold water over it. Skin each pod by squeezing them gently, then transfer the skinned beans to a bowl.

3. Add some feta cheese and mint leaves, then drizzle some oil on top. Season it with salt and pepper. Toss everything together.

4. Add the salad greens, tomatoes, lemon juice, and the remaining olive oil.

5. Toast the baguette on both sides. Make sure that they are brown and crispy. Spoon cheese and bean mixture over the toast serve everything with the season salad greens on the side.

Avocado Toast

Are you always rushing in the morning? Do you not have time for anything more than a toast? Well, why not make your toast more interesting by having avocados on them? Avocados are healthy and rich in healthy fat and fiber, so your breakfast is going to be packed.

Calories	Protein	Carbohydrates	Fat
200	5	18	13

Ingredients:

- 1 avocado

- 1 slice whole-grain bread, toasted

- 1 tsp lemon juice

- ½ tsp extra virgin olive oil

- 1 pinch red pepper flakes

- salt and pepper, to taste

Instructions:

1. In a bowl, bring together the lemon juice and avocado. Mash the avocado with a fork. Season this with salt and pepper.

2. Toast a piece of whole wheat bread. Spread some avocado on the toast.

3. Drizzle it with olive oil and top it with red pepper flakes.

Skillet Poached Eggs

Also known as Shakshuka and it is s traditional Mediterranean dish with the eggs as the most prominent feature. It is a delicious breakfast dish that will surely wake you up and kickstart your day in the right direction.

Calories	Protein	Carbohydrates	Fat
259	12	23	13.5

Ingredients:

- 1 oz feta cheese, crumbled

- 2 tbsp chives, chopped

- 4 eggs

- 3 cloves garlic, chopped

- 2 tbsp extra-virgin olive oil

- 1 cup onion, chopped

- 1 tsp oregano, chopped

- 1 tbsp fresh oregano

- 1 cup red bell pepper, chopped

- 1 can tomatoes, crushed

- 2 tsp red wine vinegar

- ¼ cup water

- salt and pepper, to taste

Instructions:

1. Preheat oven to 175ºC

2. In a cast-iron skillet, heat oil and sauté the onion and bell pepper until the onions are translucent. Add the garlic and let it sauté for about 2 minutes.

3. Add ¼ cup water, red wine vinegar, salt, and crushed tomatoes. Let things simmer until the sauce thickens or about 10 minutes. Add the feta cheese.

4. Create 4 indentations along the surface of the sauce using the back of the spoon then break one egg each. Season the eggs with black pepper. Transfer the

skillet into the oven and let things bake until the egg whites are cooked, or about 12 minutes.

5. Sprinkle oregano and chives before serving.

Brie & Bacon Omelet Wedges

These Spanish-style frittatas are the perfect breakfast partner. They are easy to make, and they're delicious—especially if you decide to add some cheese to bring some fun on your breakfast plate.

Calories	Protein	Carbohydrates	Fat
395	25	3	31

Ingredients:

- 100g brie, sliced

- 1 bunch chives, chopped

- 1 cucumber, seeded and halved

- 6 eggs, lightly beaten

- 200g radish, quartered

- 200g smoked lardons

- 1 tsp Dijon mustard

- 2 tbsp olive oil

- 1 tsp red wine vinegar

- pepper, to taste

Instructions:

1. Preheat the grill to medium heat

2. In a small pan, heat oil and fry the lardons until they are golden brown and crispy. Dry and drain it on a kitchen towel.

3. In a nonstick pan, heat some oil. Bring together the eggs, fried lardon, and chives. Season it with black pepper. Mix everything well together and then pour it into the pan.

4. Let everything cook then add the brie on top. Let things grill until they are nice and golden. Add the vinegar, mustard and remaining oil.

5. Cut the egg into wedges and toss the cucumber and radishes into the pan before serving it.

Overnight Oats

As the name suggests, overnight oats are breakfast oats that you prepare ahead of time or the night before. You do this, so you do not have to rush in the morning. But also you do this because by doing this you allow the flavors to mix well, so they're perfect when you have it in the morning. Tale note, this recipe is relatively basic, but feel free to spice it up with various toppings. You can put avocado, blueberries, cherries, pumpkin, banana, raspberries, peaches, mango, apples, and so many others. Do not limit yourself.

Calories	Protein	Carbohydrates	Fat
258	12	34	8.7

Ingredients:

- 1 tbsp chia seeds

- 1 tbsp flaxseed meal

- 1 ¼ cup nut milk

- 1 cup rolled oats

- 1/8 tsp salt

- ½ cup Greek yogurt

Instructions:

1. In a bowl, bring together all the ingredients. Make sure to mix well.

2. Store it in the refrigerator overnight.

3. In the morning, top it with your favorite fruits (or savory ingredient, if you must)

Chickpea and Cucumber Morning Bowl

Fancy some salad this breakfast? This fresh salad is more enjoyable when topped with a beautiful and runny fried egg. The textures provided by the different ingredients are interesting—they will surely party in your mouth.

Calories	Protein	Carbohydrates	Fat
365	19	28	15.6

Ingredients:

- 2 tbsp feta cheese, crumbled

- ½ can chickpeas, drained

- ½ cup cucumber, sliced

- 2 tsp dill, chopped

- 2 eggs

- 1 ½ tsp extra virgin olive oil

- 2 tbsp roasted red bell peppers, slivered

- 1 ½ tsp red wine vinegar

- salt and pepper, to taste

Instructions:

1. In a bowl, bring together the olive oil and red wine vinegar. Season this with salt and pepper.

2. Add the olives, bell peppers, and chickpeas. Toss everything together to let the flavors combine.

3. In a skillet, heat oil and fry two eggs. Set it aside.

4. Transfer the salad to a bowl. Arrange the cucumber slices and lay the fried eggs on top of the salad. Finally, sprinkle the chopped dill and cheese before serving.

Egg Muffins with Ham Filling

When you think of breakfast, you think of eggs, and this muffin is the perfect breakfast partner because each satisfying bite is like a spoonful of morning goodness. It's delicious and healthy, so that it will set you up properly for your day.

Calories	Protein	Carbohydrates	Fat
109	9.3	1.8	6.7

Ingredients:

- 1 pinch basil, for garnish

- ¼ cup feta cheese, crumbled

- 5 eggs

- 9 slices deli ham

- 1 ½ tbsp pesto sauce

- ½ cup roasted red peppers

- 1/3 cup spinach, minced

- salt and pepper, to taste

Instructions:

1. Preheat oven to 200°C. Grease a muffin tin.

2. Lay a slice of ham on the muffin tin. Make sure to cover all sides of the muffin.

3. Add roasted red peppers into the ham muffins cups and then add a tablespoon of spinach on top of the peppers.

4. Add ½ tbsp feta cheese on top of the spinach and peppers.

5. In a bowl, whisk the eggs. Season with salt and pepper, then divide the eggs into the muffin tins. Pop the tins into the oven and let things bake until the eggs are nice and puffy or about 15 minutes.

6. Carefully remove the ham muffins from the tin and garnish it with pesto sauce, basil, and the remaining roasted red peppers.

Scrambled Eggs with Spinach and Raspberries

How about a sweet and savory treat for breakfast? Some people like something salty for breakfast, but other people look for something sweet. What if you desire both? This simple egg recipe will satisfy both cravings so that you can start your day correctly. It is rich in protein and fiber but is also quite delicious.

Calories	Protein	Carbohydrates	Fat
296	18	21	16

Ingredients:

- 1 slice toasted whole-grain bread

- 1 tsp canola oil

- 2 eggs, beaten

- ½ cup raspberries

- 1 ½ cups baby spinach

- salt and pepper, to taste

Instructions:

1. In a skillet, heat oil and cook the spinach until they become wilted. Set this aside on a plate.

2. Wipe the skillet clean and add the eggs. Add the spinach. Season it with salt and pepper.

3. Arrange the breakfast toast. Lay a bed of spinach and egg. Then top everything with raspberries.

Salads

Salads make meals enjoyable because it can turn a simple dish to a whole new level when paired with an exciting salad. It can be enjoyed as a side or a light meal, depending on what you're craving.

Mediterranean Dishes are proud of the way they creatively handle vegetables. The salads in this creation are full of fantastic character and excellent flavors.

Farro Salad

Farro is a grain product, and it's not very famous, but its got a nutty characteristic smell that is going to bring so much flavor to any dish. This salad recipe is so amazing. You can make it well ahead of time, then store it in the fridge for future use.

Calories	Protein	Carbohydrates	Fat
365	13	43	5

Ingredients:

Salad

- 2 ½ cups vegetable broth

- ¾ cup feta cheese, crumbled

- 1 can chickpeas, drained

- 1 cucumber, chopped

- 1 ½ cup pearled farro

- 1 tbsp olive oil

- ½ onion, sliced

- 2 cups baby spinach, chopped

- 1-pint cherry tomatoes halved

- 1 ¼ cups water

Dressing

- 2 tbsp lemon juice

- 1 tbsp honey

- ¼ cup olive oil

- ¼ tsp oregano

- 1 pinch red pepper flakes

- ¼ tsp salt

- 1 tbsp red wine vinegar

Instructions:

1. In a saucepan, heat the oil. Add the farro and cook it for about a minute. Make sure to stir it regularly as you cook.

2. Add water and broth, then let things heat until it boils. Reduce the heat and let things simmer until the farro is tender or about 30 minutes. Drain the water and transfer the farro into a bowl.

3. Add the spinach and toss them together. Let it cool for about 20 minutes.

4. Add the cucumber, onions, tomatoes, pepper, chickpeas, and feta cheese. Toss it well so that it is adequately mixed. Set this aside and make the dressing.

5. In a small bowl, bring all the dressing ingredients together, and mix it well together until you achieve a smooth consistency.

6. Pour it to the bowl of salad and toss everything well. Season it with salt and red pepper to taste.

Chickpea and Zucchini Salad

Here's an easy salad dish with a simple acidic dressing that will complement with subtle tastes of the vegetables.

Calories	Protein	Carbohydrates	Fat
258	5.6	19	18.5

Ingredients:

- ¼ cup balsamic vinegar

- 1/3 cup basil leaves, chopped

- 1 tbsp capers, drained and chopped

- ½ cup feta cheese, crumbled

- 1 can chickpeas, drained

- 1 clove garlic, minced

- ½ cup Kalamata olives, chopped

- 1/3 cup olive oil

- ½ cup sweet onion, chopped

- ½ tsp oregano

- 1 pinch red pepper flakes, crushed

- ¾ cup red bell pepper, chopped

- 1 tbsp rosemary, chopped

- 2 cups zucchini, diced

- salt and pepper, to taste

Instructions:

1. In a large salad bowl, mix the vegetables and coat them thoroughly.

2. Serve this at room temperature. But for better results, pop the salad bowl into the refrigerator to chill it for a couple of hours before serving it, to allow the flavors to combine.

Artichoke Provencal Salad

Artichoke is very nutritious and delicious. This salad does not seem so much, but it gives more than meets the eye. The flavors are exciting, and they're easy to prepare.

Calories	Protein	Carbohydrates	Fat
147	4	18	7.5

Ingredients:

- 9 oz artichoke hearts

- 1 tsp basil, chopped

- 2 cloves garlic, chopped

- 1 strip lemon zest

- 1 tbsp olives, chopped

- 1 tbsp olive oil

- ½ onion, chopped

- 1 pinch, ½ tsp salt

- 2 tomatoes, chopped

- 3 tbsp water

- ½ cup white wine

- salt and pepper, to taste

Instructions:

1. In a skillet, heat oil. Sauté the onion and garlic. Cook until the onions are translucent. Season it with a pinch of salt.

2. Pour the white wine and let things simmer until the wine is reduced in half.

3. Add the chopped tomatoes, artichoke hearts, and water. Let things simmer and then add the lemon zest and about ½ tsp salt. Cover it and let things cook for about 6 minutes.

4. Add the olives and basil. Season it with salt and pepper, to taste. Mix well, and enjoy it!

Bulgur Salad

Bulgur is of Arabic origin and is a cereal food made from wheat and groat. It is healthy, and with this recipe, it is delicious.

Calories	Protein	Carbohydrates	Fat
386	9	55	5

Ingredients:

- 2 cups bulgur

- 1 tbsp butter

- 1 cucumber, chunks

- ¼ cup dill

- ¼ cup black olives, halved

- 1 tbsp, 2 tsp olive oil

- 4 cups water

- 2 tsp red wine vinegar

- salt, to taste

Instructions:

1. In a saucepan, toast the bulgur on combined butter and olive oil. Let things cook until the bulgur has turned golden, and it begins to crack.

2. Add water and season it with salt. Cover everything and let it simmer for about 20 minutes, or until the bulgur is tender.

3. In a bowl, combine the chunks of cucumber with olive oil, dill, red wine vinegar, and black olives. Mix everything well together.

4. Combine the cucumber and the bulgur. Toss it well.

Falafel Salad Bowl

This ultimate Mediterranean Bowl has everything you will want in a delicious and healthy dish. It's got an assortment of vegetables, as well as vegan falafels, so every bite you take is truly memorable. Cook the falafel well enough, and you can enjoy the characteristic crunch. The variety in texture and flavor will be so impressive—every bite is going to be memorable.

This recipe makes use of ready-made falafels and hummus, but feel free to make your own if you want to tackle that.

Calories	Protein	Carbohydrates	Fat
561	18.5	60.1	30.7

Ingredients

- 1 tbsp chili garlic sauce

- 1 tbsp garlic dill sauce

- 1 pack vegan falafels

- 1 can hummus

- 2 tbsp lemon juice

- 1 tbsp kalamata olives, pitted

- 1 tbsp extra virgin olive oil

- ¼ cup onion, diced

- 2 cups parsley, chopped

- 2 cups pita chips

- 1 pinch salt

- 1 tbsp tahini sauce

- ½ cup tomato, diced

Instructions:

1. Cook the ready-made falafel. Set it aside.

2. Prepare the salad. In a large bowl, bring together the parsley, onion, tomato, lemon juice, olive oil, and salt. Toss everything well and set it aside.

3. Transfer everything into serving bowls. Add parsley, then top it with hummus, falafels, and hummus.

4. Drizzle the bowl with tahini sauce, chili garlic sauce, and garlic dill sauce.

5. Before serving, add the lemon juice and toss the salad well enough.

6. Serve it with pita bread, on the side.

Easy Greek Salad

A classic Greek salad recipe that you can easily prepare if you're on-the-go and have little time. Toss the ingredients and enjoy every delicious spoonful. It is nutritious and fantastic.

Calories	Protein	Carbohydrates	Fat
292	6	12	35

Ingredients:

- 4 oz Greek feta cheese, cubed

- 5 cucumbers, sliced lengthwise

- 1 tsp honey

- 1 lemon, juiced and zested

- 1 cup kalamata olives, pitted and halved

- ¼ cup extra virgin olive oil

- 1 onion, sliced

- 1 tsp oregano

- 1 pinch fresh oregano (for topping)

- 12 tomatoes, quartered

- ¼ cup red wine vinegar

- salt and pepper, to taste

Instructions:

1. In a bowl, soak the onions in salted water for as long as 15 minutes

2. In a large bowl, bring together the honey, lemon juice, lemon zest, oregano, salt, and pepper. Mix everything.

3. Gradually add the olive oil, whisking as you do, until the oil emulsifies.

4. Add the olives and tomatoes. Toss it thoroughly.

5. Add the cucumbers

6. Drain the soaked onions of the saltwater and add it to the salad mixture.

7. Top the salad with fresh oregano and feta cheese. Drizzle with olive oil and season it with pepper, to taste.

Arugula Salad with Fig and Walnuts

Are you fantasizing about a fancy salad?

Calories	Protein	Carbohydrates	Fat
403	13	35	24

Ingredients:

- 5 oz arugula

- 1 carrot, shaved

- 1/8 tsp cayenne pepper

- 3 oz goat cheese, crumbled

- 1 can unsalted chickpeas, drained

- ½ cup dried figs, quartered

- 1 tsp honey

- 3 tbsp olive oil

- 2 tsp balsamic vinegar

- ½ cup walnuts, halved

- salt, to taste

Instructions:

1. Preheat oven to 175°C

2. On a baking sheet, bring together the walnuts, 1 tbsp olive oil, cayenne pepper, and 1/8 tsp salt. Pop the sheet into the oven and let things bake until the walnuts are a nice golden brown. Set it aside when done.

3. In a bowl, bring together the honey, balsamic vinegar, 2 tbsp oil, and ¾ tsp salt. Whish everything together.

4. In a large bowl, bring together the arugula, carrot, and figs. Add the walnuts and goat cheese on top and then drizzle it with the honey balsamic dressing. Make sure to coat everything well enough.

Cauliflower Salad in Tahini Dressing

A healthy and delicious salad--it will bring various textures and flavor in your mouth. This recipe requires you to make the cauliflower rice on your own, but if you want to skip this part, you can quickly get store-bought riced cauliflower from the grocery to save time and effort. Otherwise, follow the recipe in its entirety and make the cauliflower rice from scratch.

Calories	Protein	Carbohydrates	Fat
165	6	20	8

Ingredients:

- 1 ½ lb head cauliflower

- ¼ cup dried cherries

- 3 tbsp lemon juice

- 1 tbsp fresh mint, chopped

- 1 tsp olive oil

- ½ cup parsley, chopped

- 3 tbsp salted roasted pistachios, chopped

- ½ tsp salt

- ¼ cup shallot, chopped

- 2 tbsp tahini

Instructions:

1. Grate the cauliflower into a bowl microwavable bowl

2. Add olive oil and ¼ salt. Make sure to coat and season the cauliflower evenly. Cover the bowl with a plastic wrap and heat it in the microwave for about 3 minutes.

3. Transfer the cauliflower rice on a baking sheet and let it cool for about 10 minutes.

4. Add the lemon juice and the shallots. Leave it for about 10 minutes to allow the cauliflower to absorb the flavor.

5. Add the tahini mixture, cherries, parsley, mint, and salt. Toss everything well together.

6. Sprinkle it with roasted pistachios before serving.

Mediterranean Potato Salad

When you think of potato salad, you think of the ranch-style mayo dressing, but this is so much different. It is low-fat and is swimming in a selection of herbs, tomatoes, and peppers. It's a potato salad like you've never had it ever before.

Calories	Protein	Carbohydrates	Fat
111	3	16	4

Ingredients:

- 1 bunch basil leaves, torn

- 1 clove garlic, crushed

- 1 tbsp olive oil

- 1 onion, sliced

- 1 tsp oregano

- 100g roasted red pepper. Sliced

- 300g potato, halved

- 1 can cherry tomatoes

- salt and pepper, to taste

Instructions:

1. In a saucepan, heat oil and sauté onions until they are translucent. Add oregano and garlic. Cook everything for a minute.

2. Add the pepper and tomatoes. Season with salt and pepper, then let things simmer for about 10 minutes. Set this aside.

3. In a pot, boil the potatoes in salted water. Let things cook until they become quite tender, or that should be about 15 minutes. Drain it well.

4. Combine the potatoes with the sauce, then add basil and olives. Finally, toss everything before serving.

Quinoa & Pistachio Salad with Currant

Grains are very prominent in Mediterranean Cuisine. Quinoa, although relatively new in the scene, has taken its comfortable place at the center. This salad is interesting. The currants give it incredible texture and taste. But feel free to substitute it with raisins if you want.

Calories	Protein	Carbohydrates	Fat
248	7	35	9.8

Ingredients:

- ¼ tsp cumin

- ½ cup dried currants

- 1 tsp lemon rind, grated

- 2 tbsp lemon juice

- ½ cup green onions, chopped

- 1 tbsp mint, chopped

- 2 tbsp extra virgin olive oil

- ¼ cup parsley, chopped

- ¼ tsp ground pepper

- 1/3 cup pistachios, chopped

- 1 ¼ cups quinoa, uncooked

- 1 2/3 cups water

Instructions:

1. In a saucepan, bring together 1 2/3 cups water, currants, and quinoa. Cook everything until it boils, then reduce heat. Simmer everything for about 10 minutes and let the quinoa become fluffy. Set it aside for about 5 minutes.

2. In a bowl, transfer the quinoa mixture. Add the nuts, mint, onions, and parsley. Mix everything.

3. In another bowl bring together the lemon rind, lemon juice, currants, cumin, and oil. Whisk them together.

4. Combine the dry and wet ingredients. Enjoy!

Soups

Soup is another side dish that you can enjoy with a meal. Often served warm, it helps to keep your stomach ready to receive a meal, and if you're feeling a little ill, a bowl of anything warm is almost equivalent to a friendly and comforting hug.

These soup dishes are easy to make and nutritious. If you're looking for something light and delicious, a well-prepared soup can be a sufficient meal or snack.

Avgolemono Chicken Soup

Avgolemono is an egg-lemon sauce made by combining egg and lemon with broth. It is prominent in various cuisines such as Greek, Arab, Turkish, Jewish, and Italian. This soup dish takes the famous Avgolemono sauce into a whole different level. It is easy to make, but they're delicious.

Calories	Protein	Carbohydrates	Fat
451	32	42	15

Ingredients:

- 6 cups chicken broth

- 1 cup chicken breast, cooked and shredded

- 3 eggs

- ¼ cup lemon juice

- 1 cup orzo

- salt and pepper, to taste

Instructions:

1. In a pot, heat the chicken stock in medium heat and bring it to boil.

2. Add the orzo and let it cook to al dente. Do not allow it to get limp and too soft.

3. In a bowl, beat the 3 eggs. Slowly add the 1 cup of hot broth, whisking it with the egg as you do. As soon as the egg is mixed correctly with the 1 cup of broth, bring everything back to the pot.

4. Add the shredded chicken to the broth and let things simmer until the soup thickens. That should take about 4-5 minutes. Season it with salt and pepper

Tomato and Lentil Soup

The beauty of lentils is the health benefits it offers. It is rich in protein, and it is very heart-friendly. With regular intake, lentils can help lower your cholesterol levels, so how about a soup recipe that will allow you to enjoy something healthy? This recipe uses tomato puree, but if you want it chunkier, you can use diced tomatoes.

Calories	Protein	Carbohydrates	Fat
260	14.7	37.9	2.3

Ingredients:

- ¼ cup balsamic vinegar (or red wine vinegar)

- 6 cups vegetable broth

- 2 cups celery, chopped

- ¼ tsp cloves

- 4 cloves garlic, minced

- 2 cups dried lentils

- 1 tbsp olive oil

- 2 cups onion, chopped

- 1 cup parsley, chopped

- 2 cans Roma tomatoes

- salt and pepper, to taste

Instructions:

1. In a pot, sauté onions and celery. Let things cook until the onions are translucent or about 10 minutes.

2. In a food processor, puree the tomatoes. Add these to the pot of celery.

3. Add the lentils and the broth into the pot and let things simmer uncovered, for about 20 minutes.

4. Add ½ cup parsley, garlic, wine, clove, salt, and pepper. Mix well and let things simmer for a further 25 minutes.

5. Add balsamic vinegar and simmer for a final 5 minutes before serving.

Quinoa Vegetable Soup

The flavor and texture combination you get in every bite is fascinating with this quinoa soup. The selection of vegetables is incredible. You would love every spoonful you take of this fantastic soup.

Calories	Protein	Carbohydrates	Fat
144	7	19	4.8

Ingredients:

- 6 cups unsalted chicken broth

- ¼ cup Brussels sprouts, sliced

- ¼ cup carrot, diced

- ¼ cup celery root, diced

- ¾ tsp ground cumin

- 4 cloves garlic, sliced

- 2 tbsp olive oil

- ¼ cup onion

- ¼ cup parsley, chopped

- ¼ cup red bell pepper, diced

- ¼ cup russet potato, diced

- 1 cup uncooked quinoa

- 1 tsp rosemary, minced

- ½ cup zucchini, diced

- salt, to taste

Instructions:

1. Preheat oven to 175°C

2. On a baking sheet, spread the uncooked quinoa. Pop it into the oven and let things bake until they have turned brown or about 30 minutes. Remember to stir the quinoa every 10 minutes so it would not stick to the bottom of the sheet.

3. In a stockpot, heat the oil. Add the onion, garlic, bell pepper, and carrot. Let things simmer until the vegetables are tender.

4. Add the broth, celery root, potatoes, and the roasted quinoa. Turn the heat up, bring it to a boil.

5. Add the Brussel sprouts and the zucchini. Continue cooking everything until the quinoa is cooked through. Season it with salt, to taste. Top it with parsley.

Zuppa Di Pesce

Pesce is fish, and Zuppa di Pesce is an exciting fish soup, which is a rustic stew with flavors that offer comfort, especially when you're not feeling well. It is a simple soup that tastes amazing. This recipe is made with fish, scallops, and shrimps. But feel free to tweak the seafood component to your specific liking.

Calories	Protein	Carbohydrates	Fat
393	56	0	0

Ingredients

- 1 cup seafood broth

- 1 ear of corn, cut into 4 pieces

- 1 tbsp Old Bay seasoning

- 1 tbsp parsley, chopped

- ½ tsp red pepper

- 1 red potato, quartered

- 4 oz scallops

- 1 lb shrimps, deveined and tailed removed

- 2 cups water

- salt, to taste

Instructions

1. In a large pot or a Dutch oven, bring together the water, seafood stock, and salt to taste. Let things cook until it begins boiling.

2. Add the corn and potatoes. Let everything cook until the potato becomes tender or about 10 minutes.

3. Add the scallops and shrimps to the pot. Let it cook for about 4 minutes.

4. To serve, sprinkle it with red pepper and parsley.

Potato Soup

This soup recipe may seem intimidating and a lot of work. However, you should not cower away from it because it is very delicious, healthy, and perfect for the heart. The flavors are incredible, and if you are a fan of vegetables, this is the best way to enjoy them.

Calories	Protein	Carbohydrates	Fat
350	19	62	5

Ingredients:

- 3 carrots, sliced

- ¼ cup Parmesan cheese, shredded

- 4 cups chicken broth

- 1 clove garlic, minced

- 2 tsp Italian seasoning

- 1 can red kidney beans

- 1 cup whole wheat noodles, uncooked

- 1 ½ tsp olive oil

- ½ cup onion

- ¼ tsp ground pepper

- 3 potatoes, cubed

- 2 cups spinach

Instructions:

1. In a pot, sauté onions and garlic until the onions are translucent or about 4 minutes.

2. Add the water, chicken (or vegetable) broth, carrots, potatoes, and the seasonings. Cover everything and bring it to a boil.

3. Once it boils, reduce the heat and let things simmer. Add the noodles and the kidney beans and bring the pot to a boil again. Cook everything until the noodles are nice and soft.

4. Just before serving, add the spinach on top.

Lemon & Chicken Soup

This soup is creamy and satisfying. The flavors complement each other very well, and this bowl is perfectly comforting, especially when you're feeling a little gloomy or down with an illness. Feel free to substitute the milk to almond milk if you are lactose intolerant.

Calories	Protein	Carbohydrates	Fat
330	32	12	6

Ingredients:

- 2 tbsp basil, chopped

- 2 cans chicken broth

- 1 carrot, sliced

- 2 cups chicken, cubed

- 1 tbsp cornstarch

- 1 clove garlic, chopped

- ¼ cup lemon juice

- ½ cup red bell pepper strips, sliced

- ½ cup long-grain white rice

Instructions:

1. In a saucepan, heat the broth and bring it to a boil. Add the carrots and the rice. Cook everything until the carrots is tender.

2. Add the chicken, lemon juice, bell pepper, and garlic. Let things simmer.

3. In a small bowl, bring together the cornstarch and evaporated milk. Add this to the soup.

4. Stir slowly and add the remaining evaporated milk by increment. Continue heating and bring it to a slight boil and continue stirring for a while.

5. Remove from the heat and transfer to a bowl. Serve with basil on top.

White Bean & Kale Soup

The most significant feature of this soup dish is its characteristic garlicky taste. The flavors are incredible, and if you are not entirely vegetarian, you should know that this comes with a sausage surprise. Feel free to accompany the soap with toast.

Calories	Protein	Carbohydrates	Fat
200	15	21	8

Ingredients:

- 1 lb white kidney beans

- 6 cups chicken broth

- 1 carrot, diced

- 1 celery, diced

- 5 cloves garlic, minced

- 1 lb kale, torn

- 1 tbsp lemon juice

- ½ tsp lemon zest

- 2 tbsp olive oil

- ½ onion, diced

- 1/8 tsp red pepper flakes, crushed

- 1 ½ lb sweet Italian sausage

- salt and pepper, to taste

Instructions:

1. Skin the sausages and tear them apart into small pieces

2. In a deep pot or Dutch oven, heat 1 tbsp oil and cook the sausages until they have browned. Drain the fat and transfer sausages to a plate.

3. Add the remaining oil to the pot and sauté the onions. Cook them until they're translucent and fragrant.

4. Add the celery and carrots. Stir them until they have browned. Make sure to scrape any bits that stick to the bottom of the pan.

5. Add the garlic and pepper flakes. Season it with salt and pepper.

6. Add the broth and cook everything until it boils.

7. As soon as it boils, turn down the heat. Add the sausage and half of the beans. Meanwhile, mash the rest of the beans and add them into the pot.

8. Add the kale and let things simmer until they become quite tender.

9. Add the lemon juice and the lemon zest — season with salt and pepper.

Shrimp, Tomato & Rice Soup

This soup is packed and is a meal on its own. It is a healthy, protein-rich meal that's filling but low in calories. Feel free to substitute the protein source, but this recipe goes best with shrimps.

Calories	Protein	Carbohydrates	Fat
456	42	53	8

Ingredients:

- 2 bay leaves

- 1 tbsp garlic, minced

- 1 lemon, juiced

- 1 tsp olive oil

- olive oil spray

- 1 cup onion, diced

- 1 pinch parsley

- 1 cup bell pepper, diced

- 5 cups brown rice

- 1 ½ lb shrimps, peeled and deveined

- 4 cups spinach

- 1 tbsp thyme

- 1 pinch salt and pepper

Instructions:

1. In a skillet, heat oil and cook the shrimps. Season with salt and pepper. Let things cook until the edges burn.

2. Lower the heat, then add the garlic and onions. Keep cooking until the onions caramelize, but make sure not to burn the garlic. Scrape the bottom to remove anything that got stuck.

3. Add thyme and keep cooking, while stirring

4. Add the broth, rice, and tomatoes. Let things simmer. Add the bay leaves then season with salt and pepper.

Cook everything for a further 10 minutes. Keep adding water the pot is drying up.

5. Once cooked, add the remaining broth. Garnish with parsley and lemon.

Pear & Squash Soup

The flavors in a bowl of pear and squash soup is a medley of flavors from Morocco and Spain. Rich in fiber and protein, every spoonful brings fantastic comfort to you. The squash, pear, and cinnamon go so well together—it can genuinely make a difference.

Calories	Protein	Carbohydrates	Fat
223	6	27	12

Ingredients:

- 2 cup chicken broth

- 1 stick cinnamon

- 2 cloves garlic

- ½ cup white kidney beans

- 4 tbsp extra virgin olive oil

- 1 onion

- 1 tsp dried oregano

- 2 tbsp fresh oregano

- 2 tbsp parsley

- 1 pear, cored and chopped

- 1 pinch black pepper

- 1 pinch, 1 tsp salt

- 1 butternut squash, peeled and diced

- 2 tbsp walnut

- ¼ cup Greek yogurt

Instructions:

1. Preheat oven to 175°C

2. In a bowl, bring together the olive oil, salt, and squash

3. Transfer this mixture to a roasting pan and make sure to spread everything evenly. Pop it into the oven and let things bake for about 25 minutes.

4. In a pot, heat oil and sauté onions until they become translucent. Add garlic, dried oregano, and cook for about 1 minute.

5. Add the squash cinnamon stick, pear, and broth. Season with salt and pepper, then cover everything and let things come to a boil.

6. As soon as it boils, add the walnuts and bean, then reduce the heat and let things simmer for awhile to allow the flavors to combine. You can leave it for about 20 minutes.

7. Remove the cinnamon stick and then run the soup in a blender to smoothen everything out

8. Add yogurt, mixing the soup as you do, and let the soup come to a creamy consistency.

9. Add parsley and oregano — season with salt and pepper, to taste.

Hummus Soup

Hummus is mostly known as a dip, but this soup transforms an already popular dish into something more spectacular and healthy. This vegetarian soup brings to life the flavors of a traditional falafel, so go ahead and enjoy it with a piece of toasted pita so you can dunk into the goodness.

Calories	Protein	Carbohydrat es	Fat
170	5	15	9

Ingredients:

Soup

- 1 bell pepper, chopped

- 3 cups vegetable broth

- 2 tbsp butter

- 1 can chickpeas

- 1 tsp ground coriander

- 1 tsp ground cumin

- 4 cloves garlic

- 1 tbsp lemon juice

- 2 cups onions, diced

- 1/8 tsp cayenne pepper

- ¾ tsp salt

- 2 tbsp tahini paste

Toppings

- 1/w cup feta cheese, crumbled

- ¼ cup cilantro, chopped

- 1 lemon, cut in wedges

- ¼ cup parsley, chopped

- 1 plum tomato, diced

- ½ cup yogurt

Instructions:

1. In a deep pot or a Dutch oven, heat butter and sauté onions, cumin, bell pepper, and coriander. Season with salt and red pepper. Let things cook for about 8 minutes or until the onions are translucent.

2. Add the garlic and the chickpeas. Continue stirring as you cook.

3. Add the broth and turn the heat up. Cook everything for a minute and then remove the pot from the heat.

4. In a blender, blend the mixture by increments, until you achieve a smooth consistency. Add lemon juice.

5. Serve with tomato, feta cheese, cilantro, parsley and yogurt on top. Finally, add some lemon wedges for squeezing.

Main Dishes

For any meal, the main dish the star, and this provides the bulk of the nutrition for the body. These dishes are not only filling and nutritious—but they are also delicious. You can have them for lunch or dinner. You can even use some of these recipes for when you have visitors in the house, and you want to serve something deliciously impressive.

Baked Potatoes and Zucchini

This potato and zucchini dish is also known as a "Briam," and it is a traditional Greek roasted vegetable dish. It is simple to prepare and delicious, especially when topped with some feta cheese.

Calories	Protein	Carbohydrates	Fat
534	11.3	11.3	28.3

Ingredients:

- 4 tbsp feta cheese, crumbled

- ½ cup olive oil

- 2 onions, sliced

- 2 tbsp parsley, chopped

- 2 lbs potatoes, sliced

- 6 tomatoes, pureed

- 54 zucchinis, sliced

- salt and pepper, to taste

Instructions:

1. Preheat oven to 200ºC

2. Prepare a large (9x13-inch) baking dish. Lay all the sliced potatoes, onions, and zucchini on the dish. Make sure to spread everything evenly.

3. Add the tomato puree, parsley, and olive oil. Season the dish with salt and pepper. Toss all the ingredients together, make sure the vegetable slices are evenly seasoned. Feel free to puree fresh tomatoes instead of using the ones in the can.

4. Pop the dish into the oven, Let things bake for about an hour, then stir everything, and leave it baking another hour, or until the vegetables are thoroughly cooked. If the veggies get a bit too dry, you may add hot water into the dish.

Roasted Salmon with Carrots, Beets, and Oranges

This amazing salmon sheet pan recipe is straightforward, but it can impress guests if you're thinking of cooking for some people. It's effortless to do. You'll be surprised by what you can achieve.

Calories	Protein	Carbohydrates	Fat
390	38	21	17

Ingredients:

- 1 Chiogga beet, sliced

- 1 golden beet, sliced

- 1 carrot, sliced

- 1 tsp fennel seeds, crushed

- 2 tbsp lemon juice

- 2 tbsp olive oil

- 1 onion, cut in wedges

- 2 blood oranges, cut in wedges

- 1 navel orange, cut in wedges

- 1 ½ lb salmon fillet

- 2 tsp tarragon, chopped

- salt and pepper, to taste

Instruction:

1. Preheat oven to 250ºC. Line baking sheet with parchment paper.

2. Dry the salmon with a paper towel.

3. On the baking sheet, lay the fish at the center and arrange the beets, carrots, onions, and oranges around it.

4. In a small bowl, bring together the oil, fennel seeds, salt, and pepper. Drizzle this oil mixture on top of the dish.

5. Pop the baking dish into the oven and let things bake until the fish breaks into flakes.

6. When done, drizzle it with lemon juice and sprinkle tarragon on top.

Zesty Lemon Salmon on a Bed of Lima Beans

This nutritious dish not just colorful; it is delicious. The zesty flavor that the lemon brings it real character and kick. The ingredients will swim along with the bed of lima beans, so it is going to be a new bite to enjoy.

Calories	Protein	Carbohydrates	Fat
340	40	25	8

Ingredients:

- 3 cloves garlic, sliced

- 1 lemon, sliced, juiced and zested

- 1 lb baby lima beans

- 2 tsp extra virgin olive oil

- ¾ tsp oregano

- 2 tbsp parsley, chopped

- ¾ tsp paprika

- 1 pinch pepper flakes

- 1 ½ cups water

- ½ cup Greek yogurt

- salt and pepper, to taste

Instructions:

1. Preheat the broiler. Line a baking dish with foil.

2. In a bowl, bring together the lemon juice with the yogurt. Add ¼ tsp paprika. Set it aside.

3. In a saucepan, heat oil and sauté garlic, pepper flakes, and oregano until the garlic is golden brown.

4. Add the lima beans, water, and lemon zest. Let things simmer with the pan slightly covered. Keep it cooking until the beans are cooked and tender. Season it with salt and pepper to taste.

5. Remove the pan from the heat and then add the parsley.

6. Add the 1 tsp olive oil, and the yogurt. Mix it slowly.

7. In another bowl, bring together the remaining paprika and season it with salt and pepper, to taste.

8. Lay the salmon on the prepared baking dish. Top each salmon with slices and season it the paprika mixture.

9. Broil the salmon until they are cooked through.

10. Arrange the lima beans on a platter and lay the broiled salmon on top of it. Top it with lemon and yogurt mixture prepared earlier.

Vegetable Moussaka

Moussaka is a dish that originated in Greece and the Middle East. It is like a savory pie, appearing much like an Italian lasagna, but it is usually packed with eggplants, potato, and may or may not contain meat. It is truly delicious. And this

Calories	Protein	Carbohydrates	Fat
341	16	36	17

Ingredients:

- 1/8 tsp cinnamon

- 3 eggplants, sliced

- 2 cloves garlic, chopped

- 2 onions, sliced

- 1 tsp maple syrup (optional)

- 1 tbsp olive oil

- 1 pinch cayenne pepper

- 12 oz smoked firm tofu

- 1 can plum tomatoes, drained and diced (save the juice)

- 1 tbsp tomato paste

- salt and pepper, to taste

Bechamel Sauce

- 2 ½ cups almond milk

- 1/8 tsp nutmeg, ground

- ½ tsp salt

- 2 tbsp potato starch

- 2 tbsp nutritional yeast

Instructions:

1. In a skillet, heat the diced tomatoes along with the tomato juice. Let it cook for about 10 minutes or until the sauce thickens.

2. Add the maple syrup, tomato paste, cinnamon, salt, and pepper. Stir it well, then take the skillet away from the heat.

3. Take the eggplants. Brush it with olive oil and season it with salt. Fry the eggplants on a skillet until they are nice and brown. Let them sit on a paper towel to remove the excess oil.

4. In another skillet, heat oil and sauté the onion and garlic. Cook it until the onions are translucent. Add the smoked tofu and let it crumble. Add the tomato sauce and blend everything well. Set it aside.

5. Preheat oven to 200ºC. Prepare and grease a baking dish.

6. Arrange the seasoned eggplants on a baking dish. Do a layer of eggplants then cover it with the tomato and

tofu sauce. Do another layer of eggplants, then add the remaining tomato and tofu sauce. Set this aside.

7. Create the bechamel sauce. In a saucepan, heat ½ cup almond milk. Add the yeast, starch, nutmeg, and salt. Heat everything until the sauce thickens or about 5-10 minutes.

8. Take the baking dish with the eggplants and pour the bechamel sauce over it. Pop the dish into the oven. Let things bake until the top is a beautiful golden brown color, or for about 25-30 minutes.

Mussels with Olives and Potatoes

Fancy some seafood today? This shellfish dish is not like anything you expect. The flavors will surprise you and bring a smile to your face, especially if you like mussels. The olives and potatoes give it a different texture—and make everything so much more enjoyable with every bite.

Calories	Protein	Carbohydrat es	Fat
345	23	30	14

Ingredients:

- 1 pinch allspice

- 4 cloves garlic, sliced

- 2 ¼ lbs mussels, scrubbed

- 2/3 cup green olives, pitted and halved

- 2 tbsp extra virgin olive oil

- 1 onion, sliced

- ½ tsp paprika

- ½ cup parsley, chopped

- 1 pinch cayenne pepper

- 2 potatoes, chunks

- 1 pinch salt

- 1 can tomatoes, diced

Instructions:

1. In a microwave-safe bowl, submerge the potato chunks and submerge it in ¼ inch water. Cover it and then pop it into the microwave. Heat it for about 6 minutes or until the potatoes are tender. Drain the water.

2. In a large pot (or Dutch oven), heat some oil. Saute the garlic and onion until the onions are translucent.

3. Add the potatoes, along with the cayenne pepper, paprika, allspice, and 1 ½ tsp salt. Stir everything

well to make sure the potatoes are coated well with the various spices.

4. Add the tomatoes and stir in 1 cup of water. Scrape the bottom of the pot if anything browned as become stuck. Let things simmer for about 10 minutes or until the potatoes are tender.

5. Add the mussels, parsley, and olives. Keep it cooking for 5 minutes or until the mussels open. Check the shells. Make sure to get rid of those that did not open.

Zesty Lemon Chicken

This chicken dish is not only healthy, but it is also very delicious. The flavors of the ingredients go perfect together, for every juicy bite.

Calories	Protein	Carbohydrates	Fat
517	30.8	65.1	16.7

Ingredients:

- 4 skinless chicken breast fillets, halved

- 4 cloves garlic, pressed

- 1 lemon, sliced

- 2 tbsp lemon juice

- 2 tbsp lemon zest

- ¼ cup olive oil

- 1 onion, wedged

- 1 tbsp oregano

- ½ tsp pepper

- 1 red bell pepper, sliced

- 8 baby red potatoes, halved

- ¾ tsp salt

Instructions:

1. Preheat oven to 200°C

2. In a bowl, bring together the lemon zest, lemon juice, olive oil, oregano, garlic, salt, and pepper. Mix everything. Set it aside.

3. Arrange the marinated slices of chicken on a baking dish. Spread the lemon marinade on the chicken slices.

4. Combine the baby red potatoes, onions, lemon slices, and red bell pepper in a bowl. Pour the remaining marinade over the vegetables. Coat them thoroughly, then add them to the baking dish.

5. Pop the dish into the oven and let it bake until the chicken is cooked.

Eggplant and Dill in Yogurt Sauce

Fancy a light but a tasty meal? It is meatless, but the eggplant is going to help fill you up sufficiently. The yogurt and dill sauce is going to be marvelous. You will surely find this interesting.

Calories	Protein	Carbohydrates	Fat
256	5	14	21

Ingredients:

- 1 pinch dill

- 3 cloves garlic, unpeeled

- 1 lb eggplant, chopped

- ¼ cup olive oil

- 3 shallots, unpeeled

- 1 tbsp walnuts

- ½ cup plain yogurt

- salt and pepper, to taste

Instructions

1. Preheat oven to 200ºC. Prepare a baking sheet.

2. In the baking sheet, bring together the eggplant, shallots, garlic, olive oil, salt, and pepper. Make sure they are properly mixed. Pop it into the oven. Let things roast for about 30 minutes.

3. Take it out, and add the walnuts, then pop it back into the oven. Let things bake for 8 minutes. Let things cool for a bit.

4. Take the shallots and garlic and squeeze them out of their skins. Bring it back to the dish.

5. Add fresh dill and top it with yogurt. Season everything with salt and pepper, to taste.

Grilled Lamb Chops with Mint Leaves

Have you ever had lamb? The best way to enjoy the richness of lamb meat is with mint because it helps bring out the right flavors. Some people are intimidated with lamb, but you shouldn't be. This dish is effortless to prepare, and you will surely enjoy it.

Calories	Protein	Carbohydrat es	Fat
238	20	1	17

Ingredients:

- 2 cloves garlic, smashed

- 12 rib lamb chops

- ½ cup fresh mint, chopped

- 1/3 cup extra virgin olive oil

- ¼ tsp pepper flakes

- 1 pinch salt

Instructions:

1. Preheat grill in medium heat

2. In a bowl, bring together olive oil, red pepper flakes, and mint. Season it with salt, to taste. Set it aside.

3. Take the lamb chops, rub the garlic all over it. Take some of the mint mixture and brush it onto the lamb pieces.

4. Grill the lamb chops about 4 minutes per side.

5. Once done, arrange the lamb chops on a platter. Sprinkle it with fresh mint and pour the mint oil, over it.

Garbanzo Beans and Spinach

This dish is also known as Espinacas con Garbanzos, is s perfect light meal or side dish. It has deep African roots and has a very interesting flavor.

Calories	Protein	Carbohydrates	Fat
169	7.3	26	4.9

Ingredients:

- ½ tsp cumin

- 4 cloves garlic, minced

- 1 can garbanzo beans, drained

- 1 tbsp extra virgin olive oil

- ½ onion, diced

- ½ tsp salt

- 10 oz spinach, chopped

Instructions:

1. In a small pan, heat olive oil and sauté the onion and garlic until the onions are translucent.

2. Add the spinach, cumin, garbanzo beans, and salt. Stir everything well together, and try to mash the garbanzos as you cook.

Grilled Salmon with Olives and Thyme

This grilled salmon dish is exciting. The foil method of cooking makes sure the meat absorbs all the flavor as it cooks. And you will love how all the aroma of the characters burst out as you open the foil. Make sure to experience that moment.

Calories	Protein	Carbohydrates	Fat
493	36.2	9.5	34.4

Ingredients:

- 4 (12x18 inch) pieces of aluminum foil

- 8 basil leaves

- 2 tbsp olive tapenade

- 4 tbsp extra virgin olive oil

- 1 pinch of black pepper

- 4 salmon fillet

- ½ tsp salt

- 1 shallot, chopped

- 4 thyme sprigs

- 10 oz cherry tomatoes, quartered

Instructions:

1. Preheat the grill and lightly grease it.

2. In a bowl, bring together the olive oil, tomatoes, olive tapenade, shallot, thyme, salt, and pepper.

3. On a foil, lay one piece of salmon and cover it entirely with the cherry tomato marinade. Fold the edges to create some kind parcel with the fish and marinade inside.

4. Arrange the parcels on the grill. Let it cook for about 7-8 minutes or until the salmon skin reaches a pale pink color. Let it sit for a while before you open them.

Cauliflower Pizza on Greek Yogurt Pesto Sauce

Who said pizza could not be healthy? This cauliflower pizza is low-carb, and it is deliciously vegetarian. You wouldn't believe it is vegan because the Greek yogurt pesto sauce is just unbelievably out of this world.

Do not be intimidated by making the dough. This recipe is not so hard, so go ahead and try it for yourself.

Calories	Protein	Carbohydrates	Fat
331	10	15	30

Ingredients:

Crust

- 12 cups cauliflower, chopped

- 1 1/3 cup, 4 tbsp Parmesan cheese, grated

- 2 egg whites

- 1 tsp, 1 tbsp garlic, minced

- 1 tsp Italian Seasoning

- Salt and pepper, to taste

Sauce

- ½ cup basil, chopped

- 2 tsp garlic, minced

- 1 tbsp olive oil

- ½ cup Greek yogurt

- salt and pepper, to taste

Toppings

- 1 pinch of basil (for garnish)

- ½ cup Parmesan cheese

- ½ tbsp olive oil

- 3 Roma tomatoes, sliced

- 1 zucchini, sliced

Instructions:

1. Preheat the oven to 200°C. Line a pizza pan with parchment paper.

2. In a food processor, put in the cauliflower and blend it until you achieve the right texture for the crust. You may tackle them in batches so you can grind them properly.

3. In a microwave-safe bowl, transfer all the cauliflower and heat it for 7 minutes. Leave it for about 10-15 minutes to allow it to cool, then drain it of excess water using a paper towel. You have to do this right if you do not want to have a soggy crust.

4. Bring the drained cauliflower back to the bowl.

5. Add Italian seasoning, salt, garlic, 1 1/3 cups Parmesan cheese, and pepper. Mix everything well.

6. Add the egg whites and blend it well, then divide the "batter" into four balls.

7. Spread the balls onto the pizza pans, allowing a ridge to form the edge of the pizza. Pop the crust into the oven and let it bake for about 30 minutes or until it is golden brown.

8. Meanwhile, bring the yogurt, garlic, and basil together in the food processor and let things run until it is creamy and smooth. Gradually add the olive oil as you continue to blend things. Set it aside.

9. Preheat the grill.

10. In a bowl, bring the zucchini, olive oil, tomatoes, salt, and pepper together — Grill the seasoned vegetables.

11. Preheat the broiler.

12. Take the crust out of the oven and assemble the pizza.

13. Sprinkle cheese on the crust. Spread yogurt sauce onto the surface then arrange the grilled vegetables on top. Grill the pizzas until the cheese melts.

Turkey Meatball Gyro

A gyro is a sandwich, but unlike your typical sandwich, the bread used is flatbread or pita bread. A delicious yogurt sauce called Tzatziki accompanies this meatball gyro. Everything about this dish is just mouthwatering. You will not regret every bite you take, so make it a big one.

Calories	Protein	Carbohydrates	Fat
429	28	38	19

Ingredients:

Meatball

- 2 cloves garlic, minced

- 2 tbsp olive oil

- ¼ cup onion, diced

- 1 tsp oregano

- 1 cup spinach, chopped

- 1 lb ground turkey

- salt and pepper, to taste

Sauce

- 4 whole wheat flatbread

- ¼ cup cucumber, grated

- 1 cup cucumber, diced

- ½ tsp dill

- ½ tsp garlic powder

- 2 tbsp lemon juice

- ½ cup onion, sliced

- 1 cup tomato, diced

- ½ cup Greek yogurt

- salt, to taste

Instructions:

1. In a large bowl, bring together the ground turkey, onion, oregano, garlic, spinach, salt, and pepper. Mix everything with your hands and form balls—about 1-inch big. Make sure they stick together well enough.

2. In a skillet, heat oil and cook, the meatballs about 4 minutes each or until all sides have browned. Let it rest as soon as it's done.

3. In a bowl, bring together the grated cucumber, yogurt, dill, lemon juice, garlic powder, and salt. Blend everything. This is your Tzatziki sauce.

4. You can now build your gyro. Using a flatbread, arrange three meatballs and stuff it with tomatoes, cucumber, and onion. Top it generously with the Tzatziki sauce to give it a magnificent kick.

Pastries & Dessert

At the end of every good meal, you want to be able to flash a satisfied smile.

Berry & Sour Cream Brulee

Close your eyes and picture this—a garden of raspberries and strawberries swimming in creamy sour cream. The contrasting flavors are sealed correctly by the richness of brown sugar. Of course, when this is served in front of you, there's always room for dessert. And rightly so, as this dish is beautiful, delicious, and good for the heart.

Calories	Protein	Carbohydrates	Fat
172	1.8	17.1	11.5

Ingredients:

- 2 cups raspberries

- 2 cups strawberries

- 2 cups sour cream

- ½ cup brown sugar

Instructions:

1. Preheat broiler. Prepare a baking dish

2. Spread the strawberries and raspberries on the baking dish

3. Spread the sour cream on top of the berries using a spatula

4. Using your hands, sprinkle brown sugar over the entire dish

5. Pop the dish into the oven. Let things bake until the sugar melts and caramelize. That should take about 5 minutes, but watch it closely so that it doesn't burn.

Red Fruit Salad in Vanilla & Lemon Syrup

Fruits are of different colors, but the most prominent color of them all is red. Red is almost synonymous with ripe and rich. It screams flavor. This fruit salad is going to be memorable. The flavors are interesting and truly mouthwatering. Be a little creative with the garnish. You can use mint, black sesame seeds, whipped cream, toasted coconut flakes or bee pollen. The topping should be something that will draw you to dessert—if the sound of a fruit salad is not enough.

Calories	Protein	Carbohydrates	Fat
235	3	58.7	1

Ingredients:

Salad

- 2 cups cherries, pitted and halved

- 2 peaches, sliced

- 1 cup raspberries

- 1 rhubarb, sliced

- 1 lb strawberries, hulled and sliced

Syrup

- 3 lemons

- ½ cup sugar

- 1 vanilla bean

- ¼ cup water

Instructions:

1. Take one lemon and take the zest with a peeler. Squeeze the lemons, until you have about ¼ cup juice. Set it aside.

2. Split the vanilla bean and remove the seeds.

3. In a saucepan, bring together the lemon zest, vanilla beans, water, and sugar. Cook everything until the sugar dissolves.

4. Add the lemon juice. Let it cool and then remove the seeds and the zest.

5. Store the syrup in the refrigerator to allow it to cool.

6. In a bowl, bring together the rhubarb and about 3 tbsp of the lemon-vanilla syrup. Let it stand for about 15 minutes.

7. Add the peaches, cherries, and strawberries. Add the syrup if you think it's drying up. Transfer everything on a serving dish. Add the raspberries then top it with whipped cream and extra syrup.

Chia Yogurt Pudding

Who said sweet desserts have to be sinful? This is a nutritional powerhouse. Feel free to use your choice of fruits, to achieve the desired flavor and colors. This dessert looks and tastes beautiful.

Calories	Protein	Carbohydrates	Fat
263	10.4	21.1	15.9

Ingredients:

- 2/3 cup chia seeds

- 1 tsp cinnamon, ground

- 2 tbsp flax seeds

- 1 cup fruits (blueberry, strawberry, cranberry, banana)

- 2 tbsp hemp seeds, hulled

- 1 tbsp maple syrup (or honey)

- 1 cup unsweetened soy milk

- 1 tsp vanilla extract

- 1 cup Greek yogurt

Instructions:

1. In a container, bring together the Greek yogurt and soy milk. Mix it well together.

2. Add the flax seeds, hemp seeds, maple syrup or honey, vanilla extract, and cinnamon. Mix everything well together.

3. Add the chia seeds.

4. Cover everything and refrigerate it for 15 minutes. Take it out briefly and mix everything well. If you think it looks too dry, feel free to add more soy milk. Take it back to the refrigerator and let it chill in there for about an hour.

Apples and Walnut with Whipped Cream Yogurt

What is whipped cream yogurt? It is heavy cream, and yogurt whipped together to give velvety goodness to a dessert like this one. The thick and fluffy whipped cream yogurt forms a perfect bed for the fruits and nuts, and in your mouth, it feels so much like ice cream, but less sinful.

Calories	Protein	Carbohydrates	Fat
315	6.4	26.7	21.9

Ingredients:

- 2 apples, cored and chopped

- 2 tbsp unsalted butter

- 1/8 tsp ground cinnamon

- ½ cup heavy cream

- 1 tbsp honey

- 2 tbsp sugar

- ¼ cup walnut, toasted and chopped

- 1 cup Greek yogurt

Instruction:

1. In a bowl, bring together the cream, yogurt, and honey. Mix everything well, by hand or with a mixer, until it thickens and forms peaks.

2. In a large skillet, heat the butter. Add the apples and 1 tbsp sugar. Stir everything until the apples soften, or about 8 minutes. As soon as it is soft, add cinnamon, and the remaining 1tbsp sugar. Coo for about 2 minutes more and then take it away from the heat.

3. Arrange everything in a bowl with the whipped cream at the bottom and the apples and walnuts on top.

Pistachio Granola with Yogurt

This simple dessert doesn't look much, but the traditional baklava inspires its flavor. But this one is made healthier so you can enjoy the same delicious taste, without feeling too guilty about enjoying something good. It is rich in protein and fiber and may be enjoyed as a dessert or snack.

Calories	Protein	Carbohydrates	Fat
320	18	36	13

Ingredients:

* 1/3 cup dried apricots, chopped

* 2 tbsp unsalted butter

* 1 tsp ground cinnamon

* 1 egg white

* 2 tbsp honey

* 2 cups rolled oats

* 2 tsp orange zest

- ½ cup roasted salted pistachios, chopped

- 2 cups Greek yogurt

Instructions:

1. Preheat oven to 175°C

2. In a bowl, bring together the oats, butter, honey, orange zest, and cinnamon. Mix everything well together.

3. In another bowl, whisk the egg. Continue whisking the mixture until it becomes frothy then add it to the oat mixture. Let this mixture dry on a paper towel.

4. Transfer everything to the baking dish and pop it to the oven. Let things bake for about 25 minutes. Let it cool.

5. Once cooled, break everything into small clusters. Add dried apricots and roasted salted pistachios. Serve on a bed of Greek yogurt.

Grape and Goat Cheese with Wheat Berry

After a filling meal, you will want to have something sweet to entertain your palate, and this simple grape dessert is going to be interesting. The contrasting flavors of the grape and the goat cheese will burst beautifully in your mouth. The texture of the grains will give it character and will make your every bite genuinely memorable. Feel free to have this for breakfast. You can prepare this ahead of time if you have no time in the morning.

Calories	Protein	Carbohydrate s	Fat
326	9	54	10

Ingredients:

- 1 oz goat cheese

- 1 tsp balsamic vinegar

- 2 cups Wheat Berries

- 1 lb red seedless grapes

- 1 tbsp olive oil

- ¼ tsp salt

- ¼ cup toasted walnuts, chopped

Instructions:

1. Preheat the oven to 200°C

2. In a baking pan, bring together the grapes, olive oil, and salt. Toss it well so that the grapes are properly seasoned. Pop it into the oven and let things bake for about 15 minutes.

3. Once done, transfer the grapes to the bowl. Add vinegar. Mix everything well together.

4. Take the wheat berries and divide them into 4 bowls. Top each bowl with the grape mixture. Sprinkle everything with chopped walnuts and goat cheese before serving.

The Rainbow Salad

A rainbow is a magnificent spectacle that usually appears in the sky following an episode of rain. It is a beautiful display of colors and when you talk about colors, this is represented well by various fruits. For this simple and healthy dessert, the choicest and most beautiful fruits are picked and prepared. It is low in calories, but it is incredible!

Calories	Protein	Carbohydrates	Fat
87	1.1	22.3	0.4

Ingredients:

- ½ pint blueberries

- 1 cup seedless grapes, halved

- 2 tbsp honey

- 2 tbsp lime juice

- 1 tbsp mint, chopped

- 1 peach, pitted and diced

- 1-pint strawberries, cut in half

Instructions:

1. In a large bowl, bring together the lime juice and honey. Mix them well together until adequately incorporated.

2. Add the blueberries, strawberries, grapes, and peaches. Toss everything well, making sure the fruits are adequately coated.

3. Top it with mint leaves

Gingerbread Quinoa with Bananas

The flavors of any gingerbread bring to mind on a special occasion—Christmas. This simple gingerbread recipe is a perfect dessert or breakfast treat for everyone during the happy holiday season when everyone is having such a great time.

Calories	Protein	Carbohydrates	Fat
213	4.5	41	4.1

Ingredients:

- 1/3 tsp ground allspice

- ¼ cup almonds, slivered

- 3 bananas, mashed

- 1 tbsp cinnamon

- 1 tsp ground cloves

- 1 tsp ground ginger

- ¼ cup maple syrup

- 2 ½ cups vanilla almond milk

- ¼ cup molasses

- 1 cup uncooked quinoa

- ½ tsp salt

- 2 tsp vanilla extract

Instructions:

1. In a deep casserole dish, bring together the bananas, maple syrup, vanilla extract, molasses, cinnamon, cloves, ginger, allspice, and salt. Mix everything well together, then add the quinoa until everything is blended well.

2. Add almond milk and mix everything. Store everything in the refrigerator, overnight.

3. When you're ready to make the dish, preheat oven to 175°C

4. Take the refrigerated quinoa mixture and whisk it to make sure nothing has settled in the bottom. Cover the casserole dish with foil and pop it into the oven. Let things bake for about 1 hour and 15 minutes.

5. Take the dish out and sprinkle the almonds. Turn the oven to broil and let things cook until the nuts have browned. Take them out and allow things cool before eating. Ll

Feta Cheese Frozen Yogurt

If you want something sweet and refreshing, especially on a hot day, this is the perfect treat. This dessert recipe is so easy to make, but it is fun and delicious. No one thinks of feta cheese as a dessert, but this will change your mind.

Calories	Protein	Carbohydrates	Fat
161	6.6	11.8	10

Ingredients:

- ½ cup feta cheese

- 1 tbsp honey

- 1 cup Greek yogurt

Instructions:

1. In a food processor, bring together all the ingredients and blend everything until it's smooth. Transfer the

blended ingredients to a full mouth container and pop it into a freezer.

2. Take the frozen mixture out and crush them into chunks.

3. In a blender, add a few tablespoons and milk or water, then blend the frozen mixture. Do this until you achieve a smooth mixture. Drizzle it with honey before serving.

Berry Yogurt Pancakes

Pancakes may not be popular for dessert, but some people would welcome a fruity pancake as an after-meal treat. Who said you could only have pancakes in the morning, right? This dish is simple and rewarding.

Calories	Protein	Carbohydrates	Fat
258	11	33	8

Ingredients:

- 2 tsp baking powder

- 1 tsp baking soda

- ½ cup blueberries (optional)

- 3 tbsp unsalted butter, melted

- 3 eggs

- 1 ½ cup all-purpose flour

- ½ cup milk

- ¼ tsp salt

- ¼ cup sugar

- 1 ½ cups Greek yogurt

Instructions:

1. In a bowl, bring together flour,baking powder, salt, and baking soda. Set it aside.

2. In another bowl, bring together butter, eggs, sugar, eggs, yogurt, and milk. Blend everything until the mixture is smooth.

3. Combine the dry and wet ingredients. Mix until it is smooth, then let it stand for about 20 minutes.

4. Fold in the blueberries if you are going to use them.

5. Grease the griddle with butter spray or butter. Heat the griddle and pour about ¼ cup of the batter and begin cooking pancakes. Let them cook until the surface bubbles. Turn the pancake and cook the other side. Set it aside on a plate and prepare the remaining batter.

6. Serve the stack of pancakes with a dollop of Greek yogurt. Top everything with assorted berries for extra flavor and texture.

Chapter 4: Your 14-Day Mediterranean meal plan

A meal plan is a meal schedule. Home cooks or home planners devotea moment of their time to sit down and lay down details about the meals they are going to have in the next week or month.

Have you ever done meal planning before? As a newbie in Mediterranean Diet, understand that it is not going to be easy to break old routines and to imbibe a whole new lifestyle. But your effort will meet more success if you are more systematic about it.

Importance of Meal Planning: Building Your Mediterranean Diet Meal Plan

If you are not used to meal planning, it may seem quite excessive. Maybe you think it' going to be a waste of your time to have to sit down and bother about what you're going to eat in the next month. But perhaps you're just not able to appreciate it yet.

Avid meal planners do this regularly because it makes their lives easier. Perhaps once you realize it's actual value, you will change your mind.

Meal Planning for Beginners in the Mediterranean Diet is essential because of the following reasons:

1. **It saves you a lot of time.** You know when you're about to cook a meal, and you spend a good few minutes staring at the refrigerator and the pantry, trying to figure out what to cook and you feel stuck? You want to whip something up, but then you realize you have no ingredients for that. It's all stressful.

   But if you sit down and build a meal plan in advance, you don't have to bother thinking about what you're going to make. As soon as you develop your menu, you can go grocery shopping and procure the stuff you need. It will save you a lot of time and effort.

2. **It is more economical.** Since you have the time to plan your meals, you can prevent excessive wastage of ingredients. You can buy components that will be

good for a few meals, and that allows you the maximize the usefulness of the food in your pantry.

The problem with mindless cooking is that you do not have a plan. You go to the grocery and you get various ingredients that you may or may not need.

3. **It promotes healthy eating.**First of all, when you're preparing your meals you get to control the recipe so you can make sure only to use healthy ingredients. Meal planning keeps things organized because you can prepare ahead of time. This way, you don't end up running out of options and resorting to take-aways or food deliveries. When you plan your meals, you take on the responsibility of choosing what to put on your plate—and you can make sure it is healthy.

Week 1 Mediterranean Meal Plan

Day 1

	Dish	Calorie Content
Breakfast	Avocado Toast	200
Lunch	Avgolemono Chicken Soup	451
Dinner	Farro Salad	365
	Total Calories:	1016

Day 2

	Dish	Calorie Content
Breakfast	Bean & Feta Toast	354
Lunch	Zesty Lemon Chicken	517
Dinner	Mediterranea n Potato Soup	111

Total Calories: 982

Day 3

	Dish	Calorie Content
Breakfast	Egg & Quinoa Bowl	366
Lunch	Vegetable Moussaka	341
Dinner	Chickpea & Zucchini Salad	258
	Total Calories:	965

Day 4

	Dish	Calorie Content
Breakfast	Skillet Poached Eggs	259
Lunch	Zuppa Di Pesce	393
Dinner	Lemon & Chicken Soup	330
	Total Calories:	982

Day 5

	Dish	Calorie Content
Breakfast	Scrambled Eggs with Spinach & Raspberries	296
Lunch	Arugula Salad with Fig & Walnuts	403
Dinner	Grilled Lamb Chops with Mint Leaves	238
	Total Calories:	937

Day 6

	Dish	Calorie Content
Breakfast	Brie & Bacon Omelet Wedges	395

Lunch	Roasted Salmon with Carrots, Beets, and Oranges	390
Dinner	Artichoke Provencal	147
	Total Calories:	932

Day 7

	Dish	Calorie Content
Breakfast	Overnight Oats	258
Lunch	Falafel Salad Bowl	561
Dinner	Garbanzo, Bean, & Spinach	169
	Total Calories:	988

Week 2 Mediterranean Meal Plan

Day 8

	Dish	Calorie Content
Breakfast	Chickpea & Cucumber Morning Bowl	365

Lunch	Eggplant & Dill in Yogurt	256
Dinner	Potato Soup	350
	Total Calories:	971

Day 9

	Dish	Calorie Content
Breakfast	Berry Yogurt Pancakes	258
Lunch	Shrimp. Tomato & Rice Soup	456
Dinner	Quinoa & Pistachio Salad with Currant	248
	Total Calories:	962

Day 10

	Dish	Calorie Content
Breakfast	Mediterranean Scones	293
Lunch	Turkey Meatball Gyro	429

Dinner	Easy Greek Salad	293
	Total Calories:	1015

Day 11

	Dish	Calorie Content
Breakfast	Pistachio Granola Pudding	330
Lunch	Grilled Salmon with Olives & Thyme	493
Dinner	Cauliflower Salad with Tahini Dressing	165
	Total Calories:	988

Day 12

	Dish	Calorie Content
Breakfast	Chia Yogurt Pudding	263

Lunch	Baked Potato & Zucchini Garbanzo,	534
Dinner	Pear & Squash Soup	223
	Total Calories:	1020

Day 13

	Dish	Calorie Content
Breakfast	Grape & Goat Cheese with Wheat Berry	326
Lunch	Zesty Lemon Salad On A Bed of Lima Beans	340
Dinner	Cauliflower Pizza	331
	Total Calories:	997

Day 14

	Dish	Calorie Content
Breakfast	Gingerbread Quinoa with Bananas	213

Lunch	Mussels, Olives & Potatoes	345
Dinner	Bulgur Salad	386
	Total Calories:	944

N.B. The meal plan prepared for you in this book is all barely 1000 calories. A tasty and healthy level to maintain is between 1000-1500 calories, so feel free to snack and consume various beverages in between.

Coffee

- Black coffee 0 calories

- Coffee with cream and one sugar 32 calories

- Coffee with skimmed milk 15 calories

- Coffee with whole milk 28 calories

Fruits (all-around 100 calories)

- 2 apples 101 calories

- 6 apricots 101 calories

- 1 banana 105 calories

- 1 ½ cup blackberries 100 calories

- 1 ¼ cup blueberries 97 calories

- 2 cup cantaloupe 106 calories

- 20 cherries 103 calories

- 2 ¼ cranberries 98 calories

- 30 grapes 101 calories

- 1 ¼ grapefruit 95 calories

- 1 ¾ cups honeydew 98 calories

- 2 kiwis 93 calories

- 1 cup mango 107 calories

- 2 oranges 90 calories

- 2 cups papaya, 109 calories

- 2 ½ peaches 96 calories

- 1 pear 96 calories

- 3 plums 91 calories

- 1 ¼ cups pineapple 103 calories

- ½ pomegranate 117 calories

- 1 ½ cups raspberries 99 calories

- 25 strawberries 96 calories

- 2 cups watermelon 100 calories

Nuts (50 grams)

- Chestnuts 101 calories

- Cashews 275 calories

- Pistachios 275 calories

- Peanuts 283 calories

- Almonds 288 calories

Wine (5 oz)

- Red wine 121-129 calories

- White wine 105-123 calories

- Sweet wine 105-165 calories

Guidelines of Building A Meal Plan

An example meal plan for 14 days is provided for you in this Chapter. You may use it as a guide to building your own. But be guided by the following tips as you stating building one:

- **Make meals flexible.** No matter how well you think you've planned for things, life is full of surprises, so you may have to deviate from the plan (from time to time). You may swap meals or change things up. You may also go out for lunch or dinner. Do not stress about it too much.

- **Check your pantry and refrigerator.** To avoid excessive wastage on food, make sure to pattern your meal plan on ingredients that you already have in your kitchen. You may explore different recipes but do not go for recipes with unique elements that you are not going to use so much of.

- **Start building your recipe collection.** As you create your meal plan, you will be gathering recipes. It would be a good thing to start building your collection. You can write them in cards and contain these in a box. You can gather clippings or print them from websites and then collate them in a clear book. What is important is you keep them in one place, so it's easier for you to plan meals.

- **Do theme nights.** If you want to start dining traditions for the home to partake in, you can do theme nights. Monday can be "pasta night," Tuesday can be "soup night," Wednesday can be "bean night" and so forth. This will be your guide in meal planning. And it will save you a lot of effort.

- **You don't always have to cook.** Contrary to what many people think about meal planning. It doesn't demand that you prepare your food all the time. Meal planning is the process of setting your menu for a given period so that you can save money and effort. Understand, however, that you can order meals from your favorite restaurants or caterers. You may even schedule dining out. Like if you usually eat out during weekends, plot that in your plans.

- **Practice batch cooking.** Batch cooking is an efficient home cook strategy that involves cooking meals in advance and "freezing" them for future use. This will save you a lot of time each day because you will set one day for you to do all the cooking so that you can freeze them.

The truth is that meal planning will be stressful in the beginning, but as soon as you get the hang of it, things will be so simple. These tips will help kickstart your new lifestyle to a good start and will help you claim victory in this endeavor. Good luck!

CONCLUSION

You are what you eat. By now, you should have decided on the kind of life you want to live because your decisions will dictate the direction your life is going to take. Maybe you have tried various diets before, but nothing worked. You should know by now, that the Mediterranean Diet doesn't just tackle the food on your plate. It teaches you to enjoy the food you eat and to do so with the company of people you care for.

Staying healthy and losing weight is not about starving yourself and all kinds of diet restrictions. What the Mediterranean Diet promotes is the lifestyle that embraces discipline through mindful eating and exercise.

The health benefits of following the Mediterranean Lifestyle is immense. It offers holistic benefits that promote optimum physical, mental, emotional, and social well-being. No other is as healthy and positively charged as this. So take what you have learned from this book and jumpstart your journey to a great beginning.

FINAL WORDS

Thank you again for purchasing this book!

We hope this book can help you.

The next step is for you to **join our email newsletter** to receive updates on any upcoming new book releases or promotions. You can sign-up for free, and as a bonus, you will also receive our "*7 Fitness Mistakes You Don't Know You're Making*" book! This bonus book breaks down many of the most common fitness mistakes and will demystify many of the complexities and science of getting into shape. Having all this fitness knowledge and science organized into an actionable step-by-step book will help you get started in the right direction in your fitness journey! To join our free email newsletter and grab your free book, please visit the link and signup: **www.effingopublishing.com/gift**

Finally, if you enjoyed this book, then we would like to ask you for a favor, would you be kind enough to leave a review for this book? It would be much appreciated! Thank you, and good luck on your journey!

ABOUT THE CO-AUTHOR

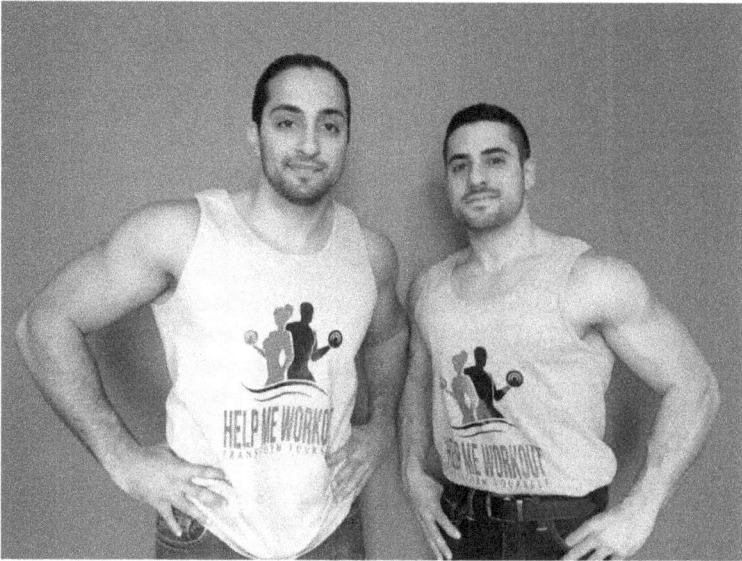

Our name is Alex & George Kaplo; we're both certified personal trainers from Montreal, Canada. We will start by saying we are not the biggest guys you will ever meet, and this has never really been our goal. We started working out to overcome our biggest insecurity when we were younger, which was our self-confidence. You may be going through some challenges right now, or you may want to get fit, and we can certainly relate.

We always kind were interested in the health & fitness world and wanted to gain some muscle due to the numerous bullying in our teenage years. We figured we could do something about how our body looks like. This was the beginning of our transformation journey. We had no idea where to start, but we both just got started. We felt worried and afraid at times that other people would make fun of us for doing the exercises the wrong way. We always wished we had a friend to guide us and who could show us the ropes.

After a lot of work, studying, and countless trials and errors. Some people began to notice how we were both getting more fit and how we were starting to form a keen interest in the topic. This led many friends and new faces to come to us and ask us for fitness advice. At first, it seemed odd when people asked us to help them get in shape. But what kept us going is when they started to see changes in their own body and told us it's the first time that they saw real results! From there, more people kept coming to us, and it made both of us realize after so much reading and studying in this field that it did help us, but it also allowed us to help others. To date, we have coached and trained numerous clients who have achieved some pretty amazing results.

Today, both of us own & operate this publishing business, where we bring passionate and expert authors to write about health and fitness topics. We also run an online fitness business, and we would love to connect with you by inviting you to visit the website on the following page and signing up for our e-mail newsletter (you will even get a free book).

Last but not least, if you are in the position we were once in and you want some guidance, don't hesitate and ask--I will be there to help you out!

Your coaches,

Alex &George Kaplo

Download another book for Free

We want to thank you for purchasing this book and offer you another book (just as long and valuable as this book), "Health & Fitness Mistakes You Don't Know You're Making," completely free.

Visit the link below to signup and receive it:

www.effingopublishing.com/gift

In this book, we will break down the most common health & fitness mistakes, you are probably committing right now, and will reveal how you can quickly get in the best shape of your life!

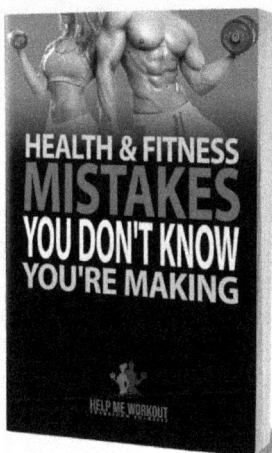

In addition to this valuable gift, you will also have an opportunity to get our new books for free, enter giveaways, and receive other useful emails from us. Again, visit the link to sign up:

www.effingopublishing.com/gift

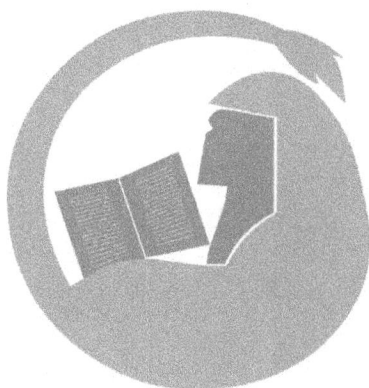

EFFINGO
Publishing

For more great books, visit:
EffingoPublishing.com

www.ingramcontent.com/pod-product-compliance
Lightning Source LLC
Chambersburg PA
CBHW060320030426

42336CB00011B/1141